The Art Gallery
of Pathology

Tim-Rasmus Kiehl, MD

Edited by Sylvia L. Asa, MD, PhD

American Registry of Pathology, 2020

The Art Gallery of Pathology

Explore the use of human pathology samples as they are used to develop art that is pleasing to the eye and challenging to the mind. For those with knowledge of pathology, histology and microscopy, the work of Dr. Tim-Rasmus Kiehl, a neuropathologist who worked at University Health Network in Toronto, Canada, will be a source of fascination.

For those who appreciate art, welcome to a new dimension of the art and science of pathology, seen through the lens of modern culture. Join Dr. Kiehl and his former Pathologist-in-Chief, Dr. Sylvia Asa, on a trip through the Art Gallery of Pathology.

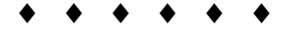

Art by: Tim-Rasmus Kiehl
Edited by: Sylvia L. Asa
Design by: Zoya Volynskaya

Printed in Korea

Preface

Pathology is the discipline of medicine that examines blood, body fluids, cells and tissues to make a precise diagnosis of disease, determine the prognosis of that disorder, and identify predictive factors that can be used to guide treatment. A significant component of the work done by pathologists involves examining tissues, including their microscopic appearance. Microscopy depends on the use of stains that allow the distinction of different cellular and tissue components based on biochemical and immunological reactions. Pathologists therefore spend their days looking at multicolored samples that have exotic patterns; each color and pattern has immense significance for the interpretation of the pathologic process being examined.

In 2006, the Pathology Department of the University Health Network in Toronto was consolidated into new space. With the move to new offices and laboratories, the staff were provided a unique opportunity to develop a new ambiance. The offices had large windows and new furniture; the labs were bright and clean, but the hallways of the Department were bare. As Pathologist-in-Chief, I had an idea: Challenge pathologists to develop pathology art to decorate the halls. After all, pathologists look at beautiful images every day; they have also been provided with high quality microscopes and digital cameras!

One of the pathologists took on this challenge with passion. Rasmus Kiehl, a neuro-pathologist originally from Germany and trained in the United States, decided to develop his creativity, and he set about to develop the Art Gallery of Pathology.

In this book, we are providing you with the opportunity to share the fruit of his labor. For those with a background in histology, the nuances of his work will be self-evident. For those who are not familiar with the scientific aspect of his work, the artistic elements are remarkable. Rasmus has been able to take tissue samples and develop them into true works of art!

We hope that you will enjoy this trip through the hallways of the UHN Pathology circa 2015.

Sylvia L. Asa, MD, PhD

Immuna Lisa

(2007)

Composed from images of various
central nervous system tumor cases
from our clinical conferences.

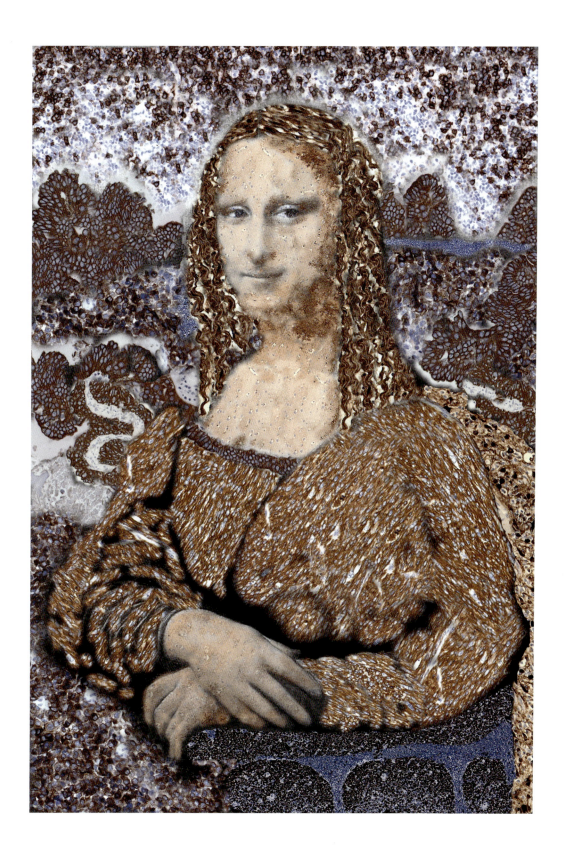

Stainhenge

(2007)

Histological stains are used to highlight
certain features of tissues.
With immunohistochemistry,
specific elements (proteins) can be highlighted
in order to find out more about
the composition of the tissue
and to improve diagnostic accuracy.
These immunostains are an ancient technique in pathology.

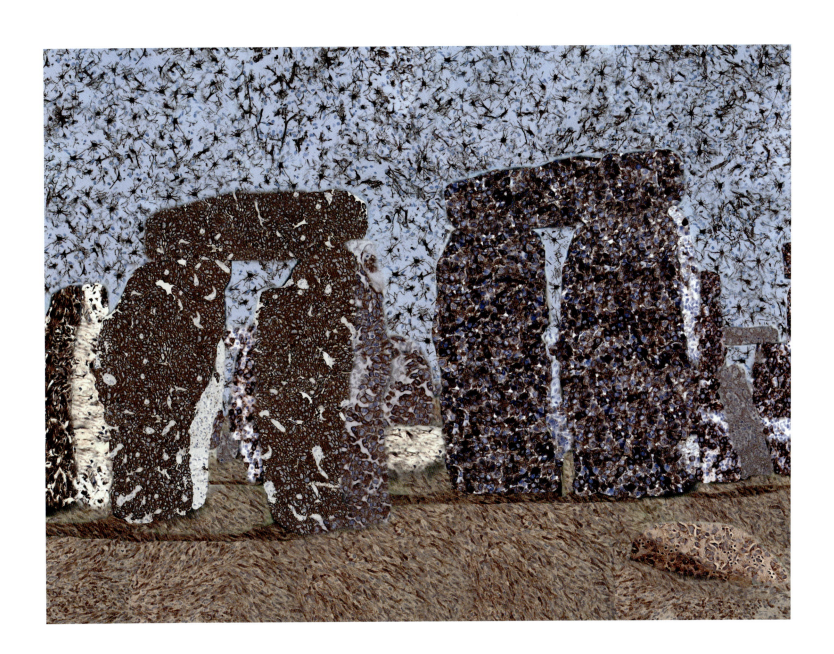

The Great Wave
of Wet Keratin

(2008)

This work was modeled after

"The Great Wave off Kanagawa" by Katsushika Hokusai,

Japan (1760-1849), created around 1831.

Craniopharyngiomas are tumors in the skull base that

tend to occur in adolescents and young adults.

While histologically low-grade,

they grow infiltratively and may be difficult to treat.

Among the diagnostic features of the adamantinomatous subtype

of craniopharyngioma are:

1) "wet" keratin
2) basaloid palisading epithelium and
3) a "stellate reticulum" matrix

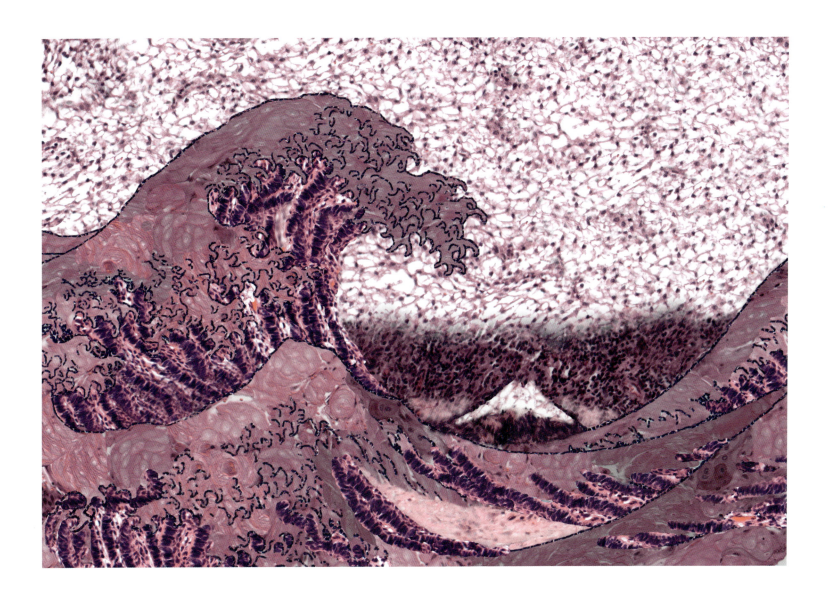

The Mighty Scream

(2006)

Inspired by "The Scream" (Skrik, 1893)

by Norwegian expressionist artist Edward Munch.

His description of the inspiration for his original painting reads:

"I was walking along a path with two friends—the sun was setting—suddenly the sky turned blood red—I paused, feeling exhausted, and leaned on the fence—there was blood and tongues of fire above the blue-black fjord and the city—my friends walked on, and I stood there trembling with anxiety—and I sensed an infinite scream passing through nature."

Histologic pictures were taken from a case of a malignant brain tumor (glioblastoma)

with a screamingly high mitotic ("mite") count.

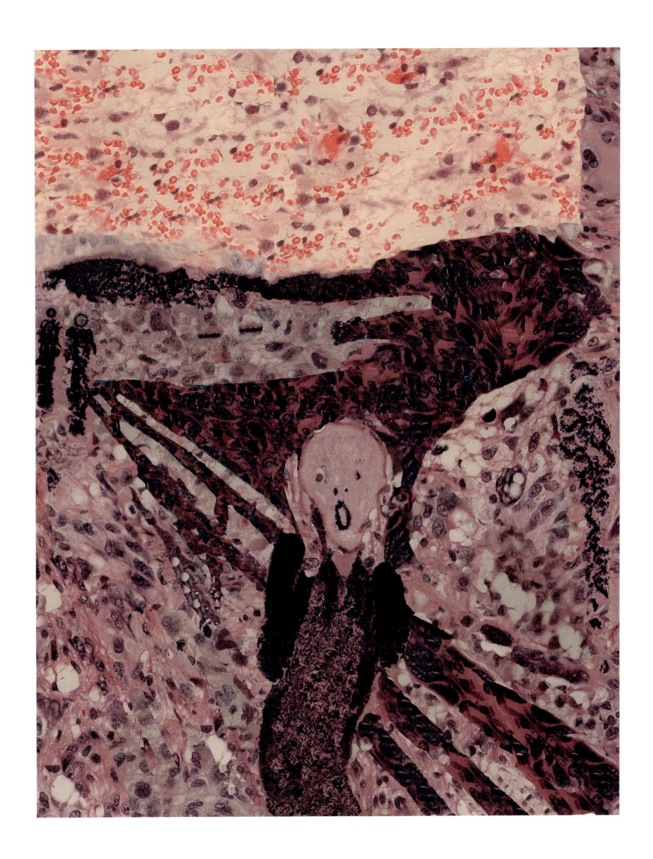

Ikaros Takes Off

(2006)

In Greek mythology, Ikaros was the son of Daedalus

Who created the Labyrinth in Crete.

Ikaros and his father tried to escape from Crete by flying

With wings Daedalus made from wax and feathers.

Not heeding his father's advice to fly

Neither too low (so the sea's dampness would clog the wings)

Nor too high (so the sun would melt the wax),

Ikaros flew too high, the wax melted

And he fell into the sea where he drowned.

The Ikaros family of transcription factors is transiently expressed

during development in the brain (basal ganglia / striatum).

This immunohistochemical stain for Ikaros used in our research laboratory

shows the onset of Ikaros expression in newborn brain cells,

just after they exit the germinal matrix.

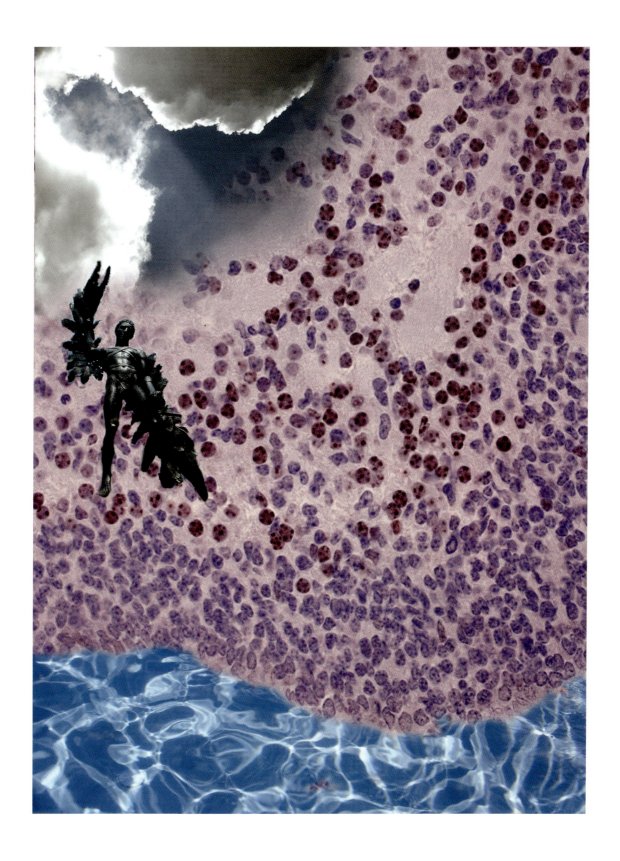

Dark Fuzzballs in Oil

(2008)

The "oil red O stain" is used to highlight small fat droplets in muscle biopsies.

Patients with lipid storage disorders may have

increased fat droplets in their muscle fibers.

In our laboratory, the solutions for this oil red O stain are prepared freshly

for each use and are thoroughly filtered.

Despite these precautions, occasional precipitates form in large oil bubbles,

often with bizarre, fuzzy shapes.

This is a composite of many images.

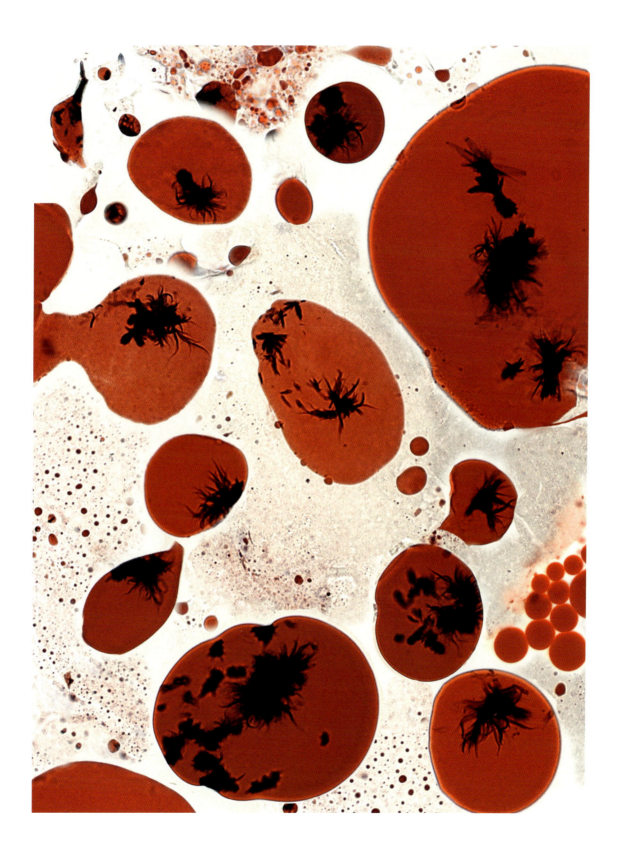

Virchow, warholized

(2008)

Rudolf Virchow (1821 – 1902)

is known as "the father of modern pathology".

One of his books, "Cellular Pathology" (1858)

is regarded as foundational to modern pathology.

This piece used a portrait photo (undated, unknown photographer).

Colors for this collage were taken from Andy Warhol's

famous artwork "Che Guevara" (1968).

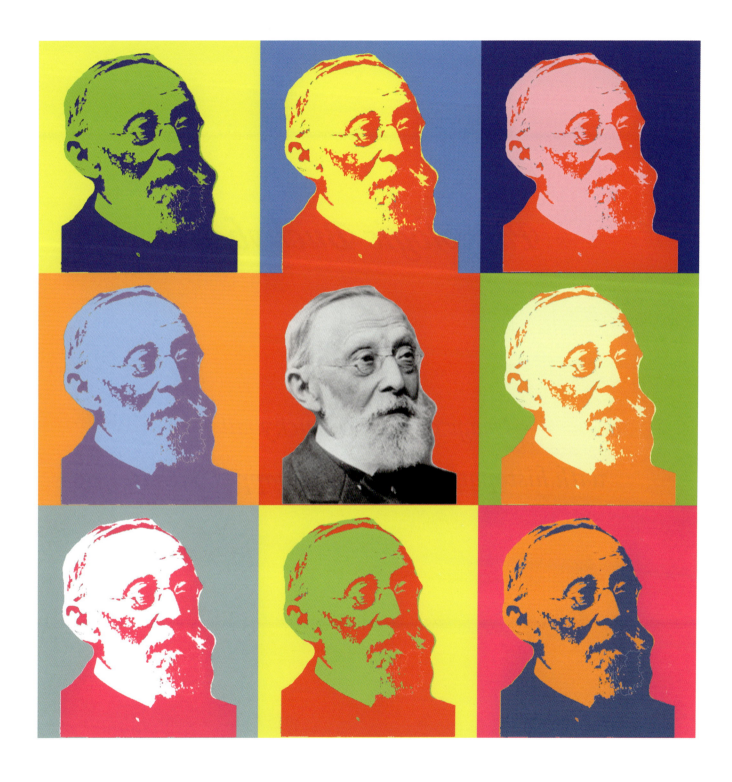

Pathologic Buckyball

(2010)

Image of a C-60 Buckyball

with histopathologic images mapped onto it.

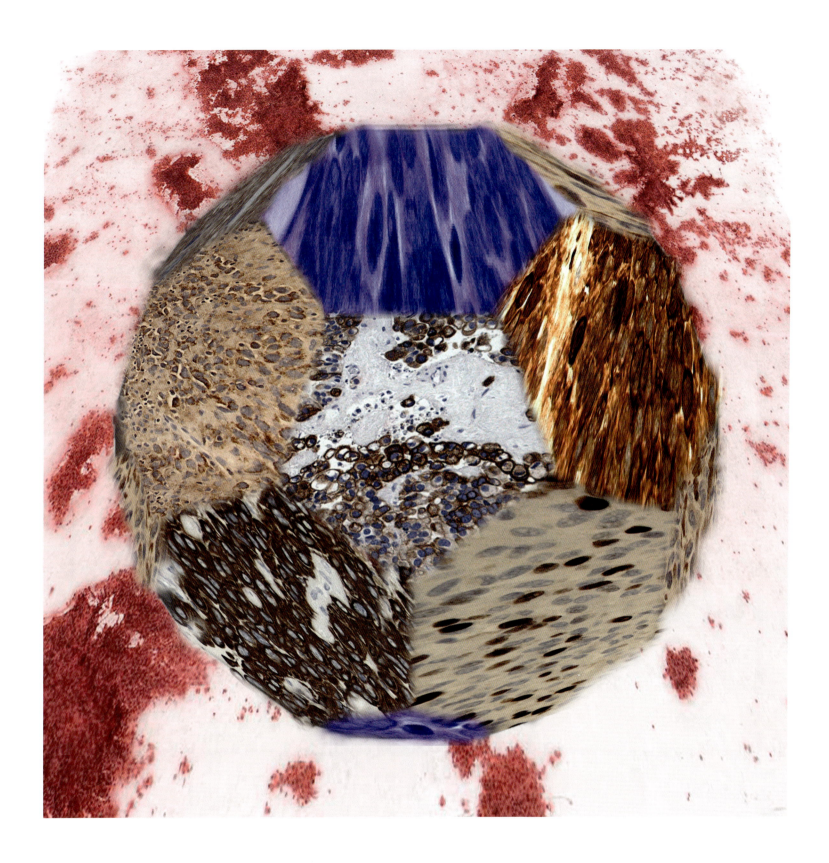

Torontonavirus

(2010)

A novel strain of hepatitis was discovered in our laboratory

by hepatopathologist Dr. Oyedele Adeyi on

electron microscopy images from a liver biopsy specimen.

We gave it the unofficial name of "Torontonavirus".

The round viral particles have been rearranged

for the purpose of this art piece.

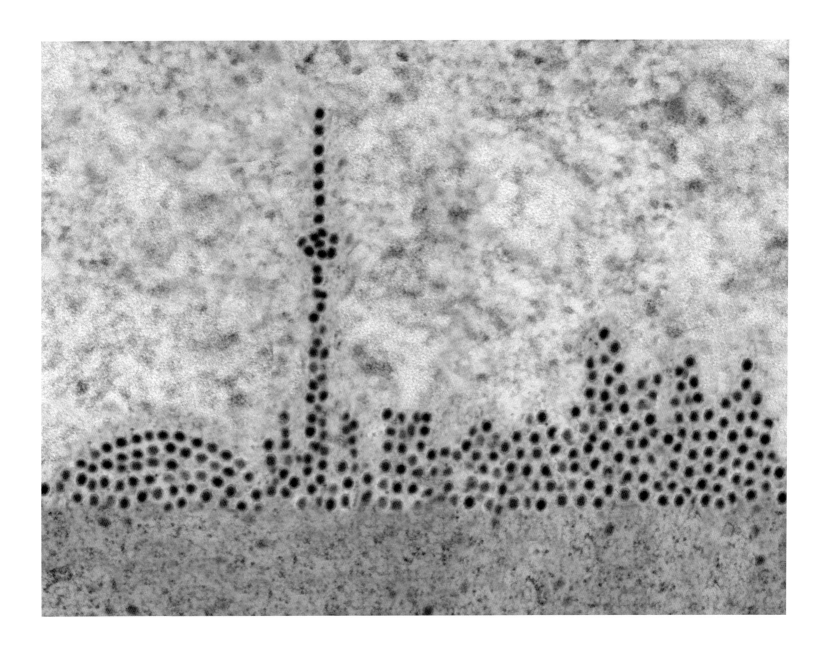

One Slow Fat Red Ox

(2010)

A popular mnemonic for the interpretation of muscle biopsies goes:

"1 slow fat red ox".

This helps us remember that **type 1** muscle fibers

are characterized by: **slow** twitch, **lipid** accumulation,

red color, and **oxidative** metabolism.

This red ox (original color, unaltered) by the name of "Herschel"

is a vibrant red Milking Shorthorn born in 2004.

It was photographed during a visit in 2010 at Tillers International,

an agricultural heritage museum near Kalamazoo, Michigan.

(tillersinternational.org)

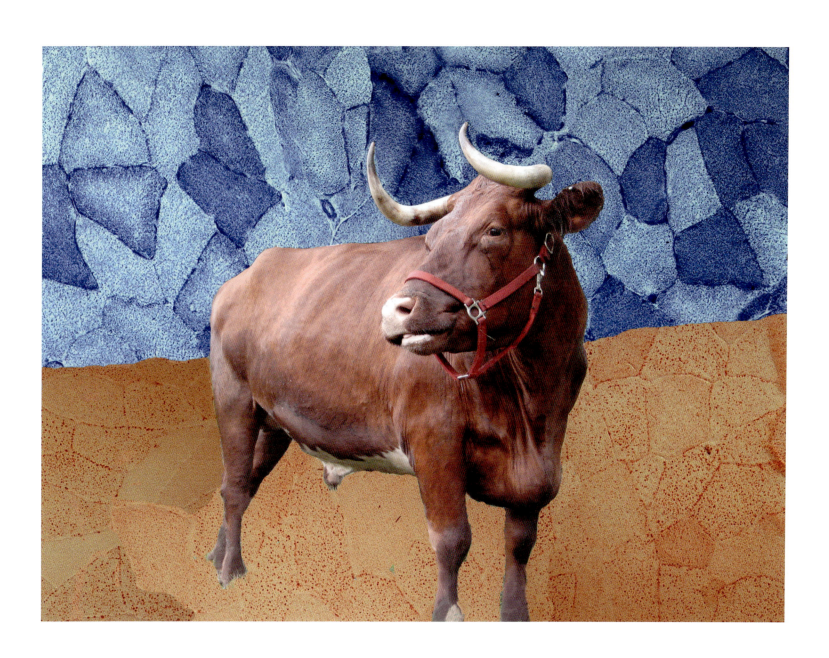

Pseudopalisading Maze

(2010)

To make it through the maze,

stay in the necrotic areas

and avoid the glioblastoma cells.

Pick up some macrophages along the way

for extra bonus points.

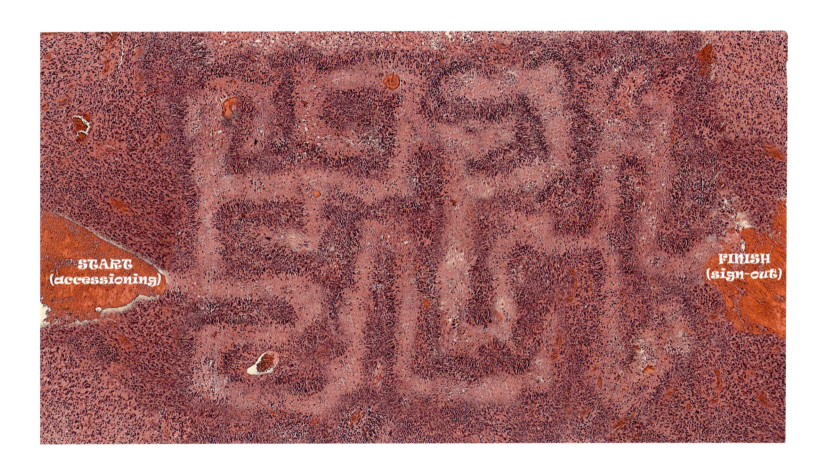

Reactive Astrocytes, Overreacting

(2010)

We received a call for an intraoperative consultation on a brain biopsy.

This also included a cytologic preparation ("smear prep").

It showed these remarkable astrocytes in their reactive

(activated, busy) state.

This is a composite of multiple images.

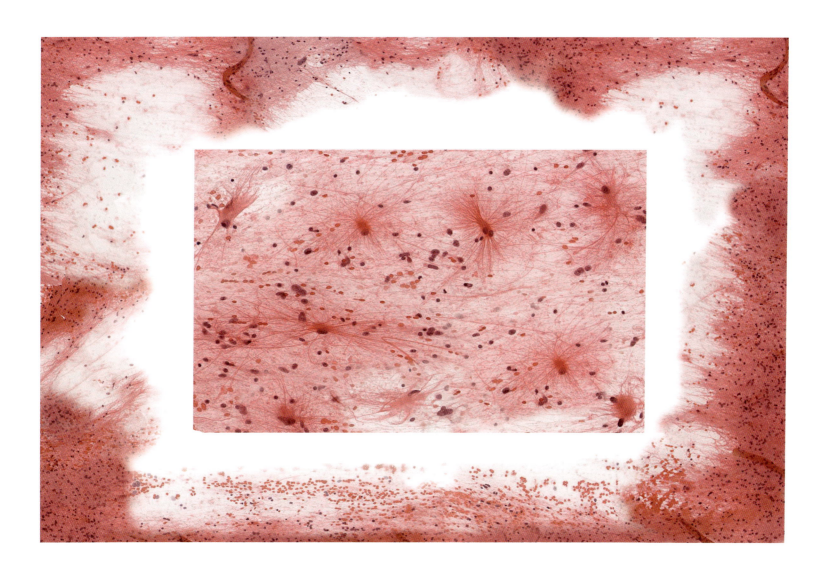

Girl with a Squamous Pearl Earring

(2010)

Derived from Dutch painter Johannes Vermeer's masterwork

Girl with a Pearl Earring

(Dutch: "Het Meisje met de Parel", circa 1665).

The expression "squamous pearls" is used by pathologists to describe a diagnostic feature in certain common cancers that occur in the upper respiratory tract and the lung.

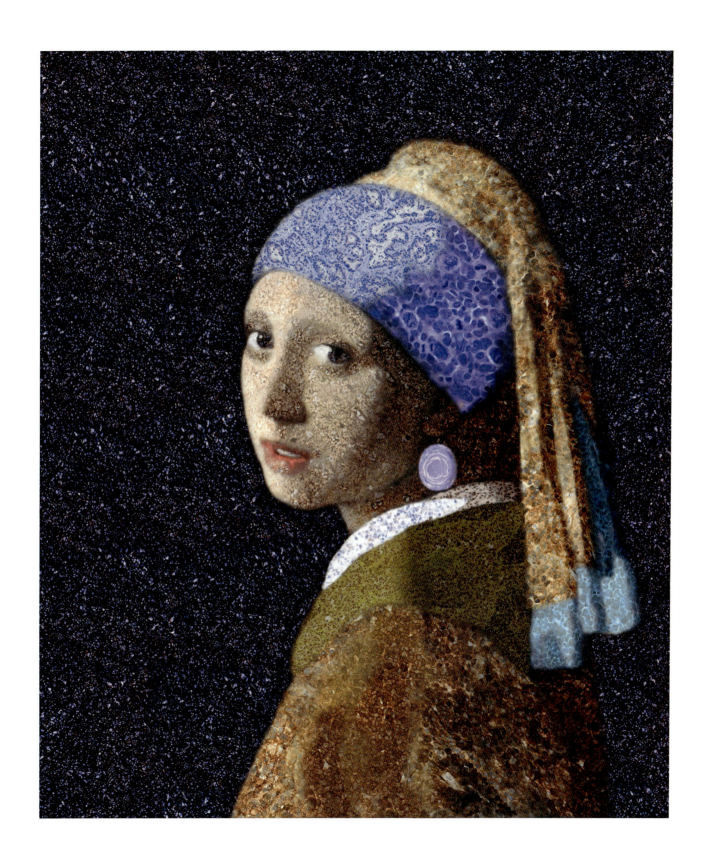

Hep

(2011)

All hope is gone.

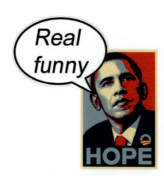

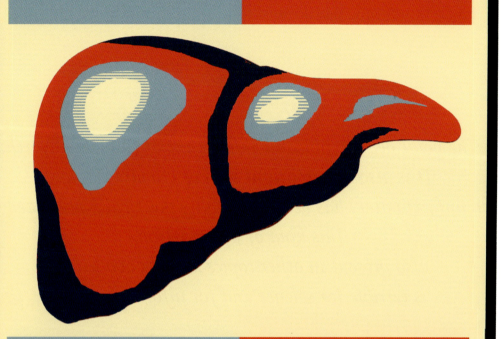

HEP

Polarized Bear

(2011)

The polar bear is an iconic inhabitant of Canada's North.
It is also an important icon of climate change,
which unfortunately has become a highly politically polarized issue.
This kind of polarization,
also present in other topics such as evolution,
is terrible for science and for informed policy.

In pathology, however, polarization is a very useful thing.
When a Congo red stain is viewed under polarized light under the microscope,
it can help us detect the presence of amyloid.
The source images for this picture were taken
from a patient with cerebral amyloid angiopathy (CAA)
in which amyloid accumulates in blood vessels,
making them brittle and prone to catastrophic events.

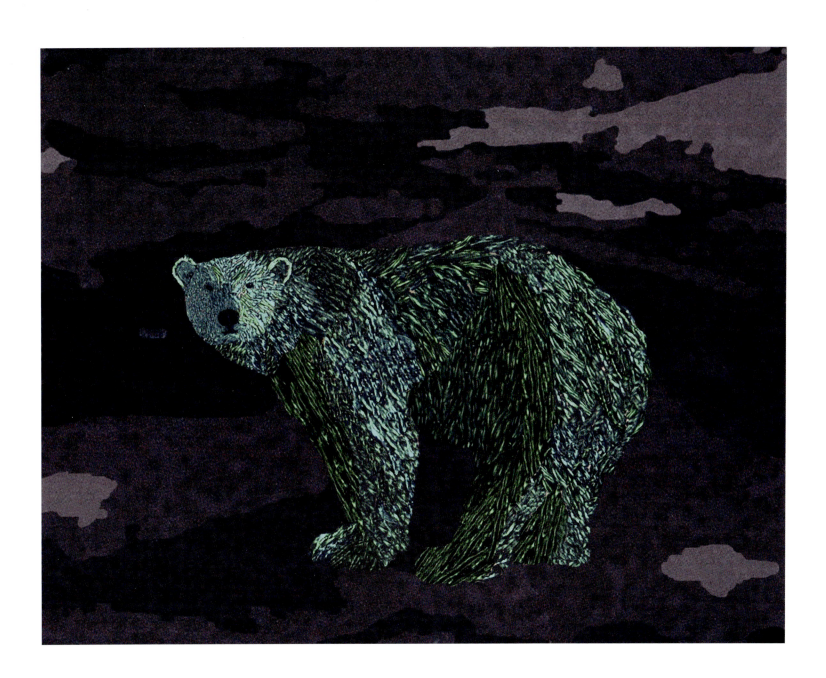

Zebra

(2015)

In Pathology, if you hear hoofbeats, think zebra!
Not just horse!

Images from this piece were taken from
A very unusual-appearing brain tumor.

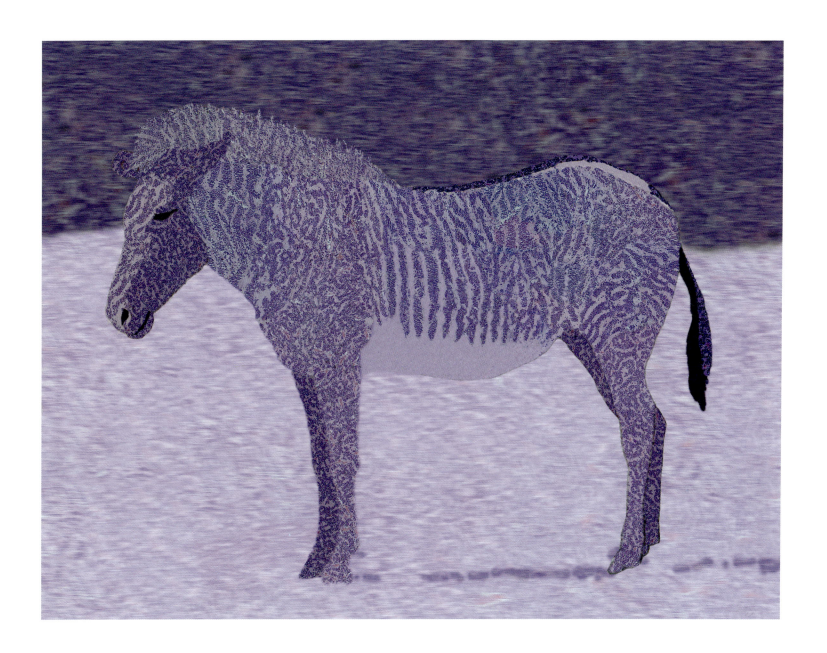

Asteroid Bodies Identified

(2011, part of "space series")

So-called "asteroid bodies",

bright-red aggregates shaped like stars,

are characteristic diagnostic features of sarcoidosis.

(images for bones and galaxies all open source via CC license)

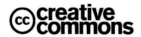

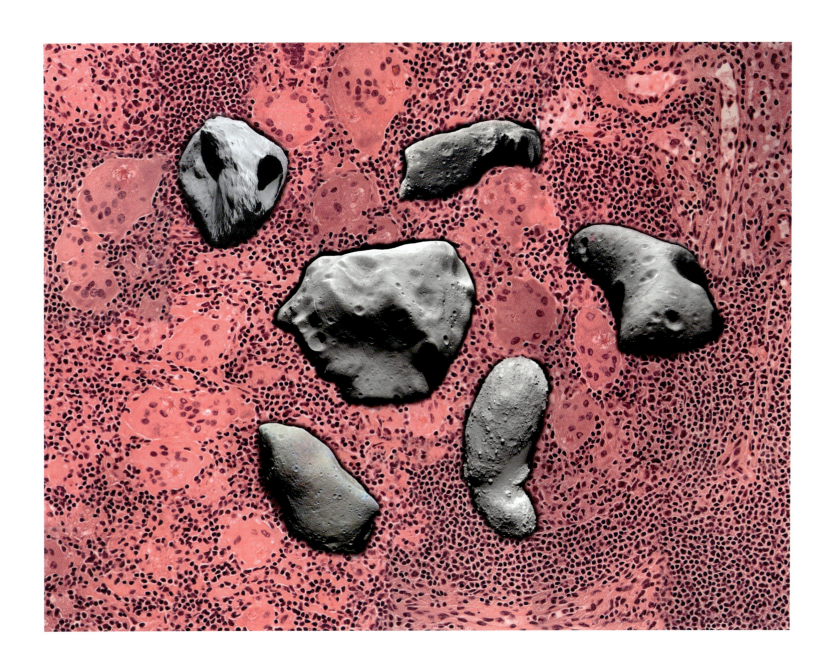

Stellar Splatter

(2011, part of "space series")

Heavy elements such as iron are not created in smallish stars like our own sun.
They are only forged under the extreme conditions of a supernova or in colliding neutron stars.
The expanding supernova remnants then seed interstellar gas clouds with these heavy elements
and at the same time condense the gas, leading to the formation of new stars and planets.
This was how our own solar system formed.
Four and a half billion years later, this same iron ended up in our red blood cells.
The red cells in this image were sourced from an intraoperative consultation
of a neurosurgical specimen (cytologic preparation, "smear").

We are deeply connected to the stars, indeed made of stars, but not in a way that
the peddlers of stupid humbug astrology pseudoscience want you to believe.
The H_2O flowing through our veins was delivered to Earth by crashing comets
from the outer solar system.
The radioactive decay heat from the heavy elements thorium and uranium
keeps the earth's core molten, creating not just the strong magnetic field
that shields us from deadly cosmic radiation
but also the tectonic activity and consequent orderly carbon cycle
that complex life on Earth depends on.

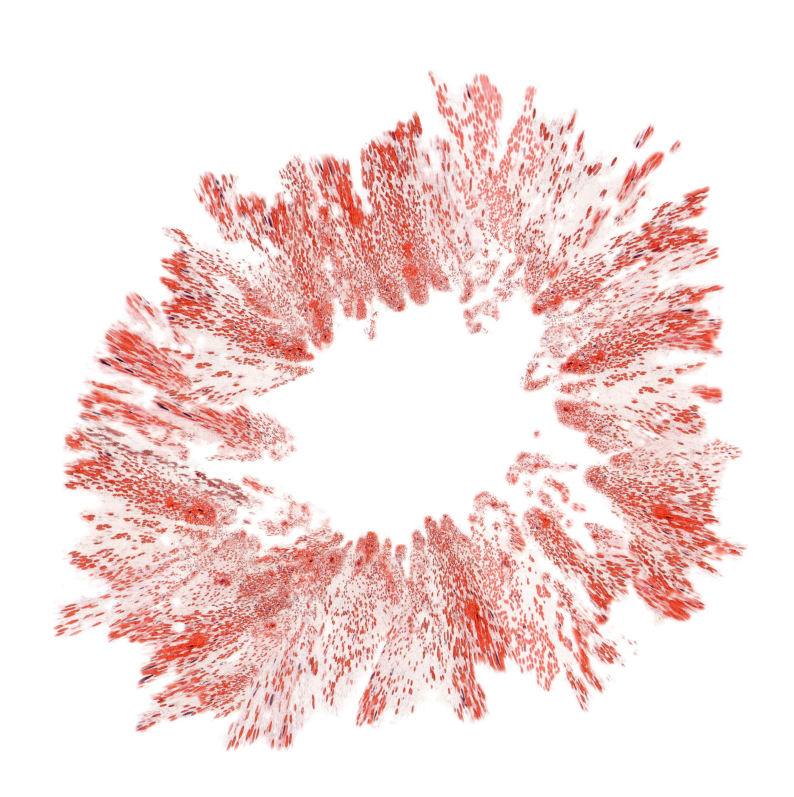

Attack of the Sphenoidians

(2011, part of "space series")

The sphenoid bone sits at the center of the skull base.
It has wings and many connection to other bones.
It is a frequent site of neurosurgical interventions,
generating pathology specimens.
A pathologist may even experience an "attack"
of many specimens at once.

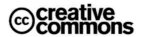

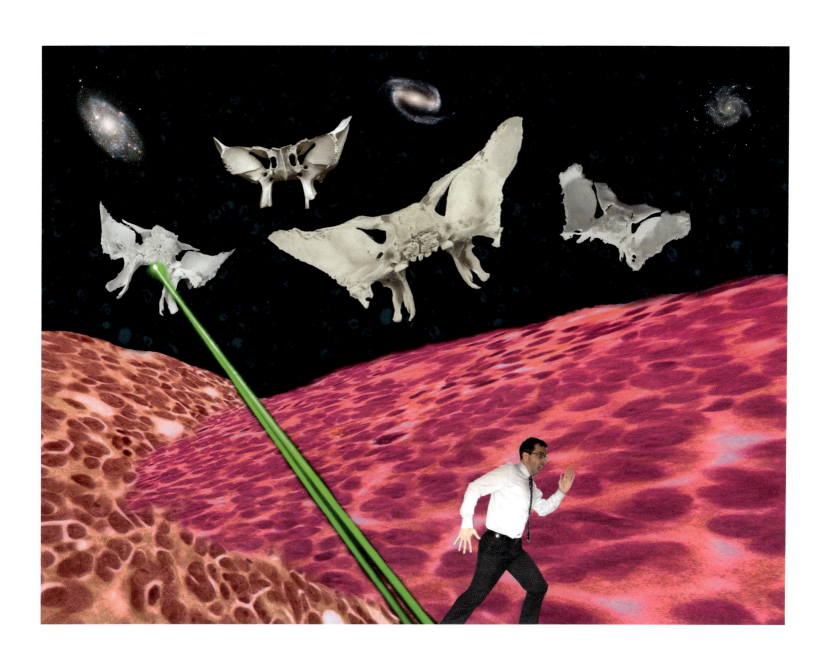

Immigrants From Another World

(2011, part of "space series")

Microglia are the resident macrophages of the brain and spinal cord,

involved in many inflammatory and immune functions of the brain.

They have a very different developmental origin than most other brain cells.

They are derived from cells in the bone marrow, so-called myeloid progenitors.

They immigrate to the brain and mature into microglia.

In this stain, microglia were highlighted

by immunohistochemistry for Iba-1.

Moon image at bottom courtesy of JAXA

(Japanese Space Exploration Agency),

taken by the Hayabusa spacecraft.

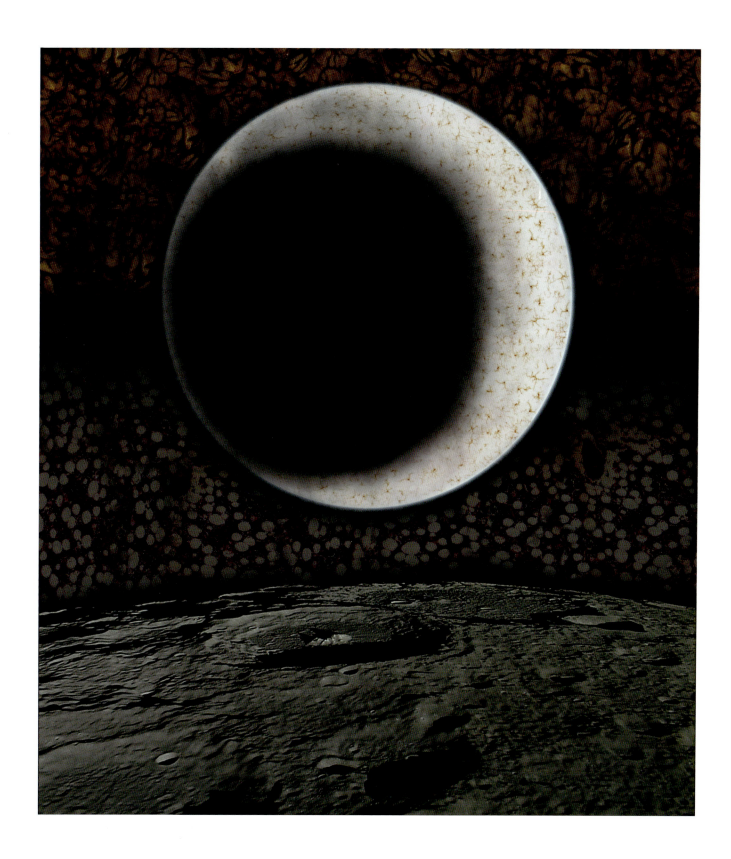

Mars in Martius

(2011, part of "space series")

As if the red (-dead?) planet needed any additional staining,

here it is painted in a stain called "Martius Scarlet Blue" (MSB),

a trichrome preparation for the detection of connective tissue,

fibrin and fibrinoid necrosis.

Source image courtesy of NASA,

taken in 1980 as seen by the Viking 1 Orbiter.

Tissue patterns overlaid.

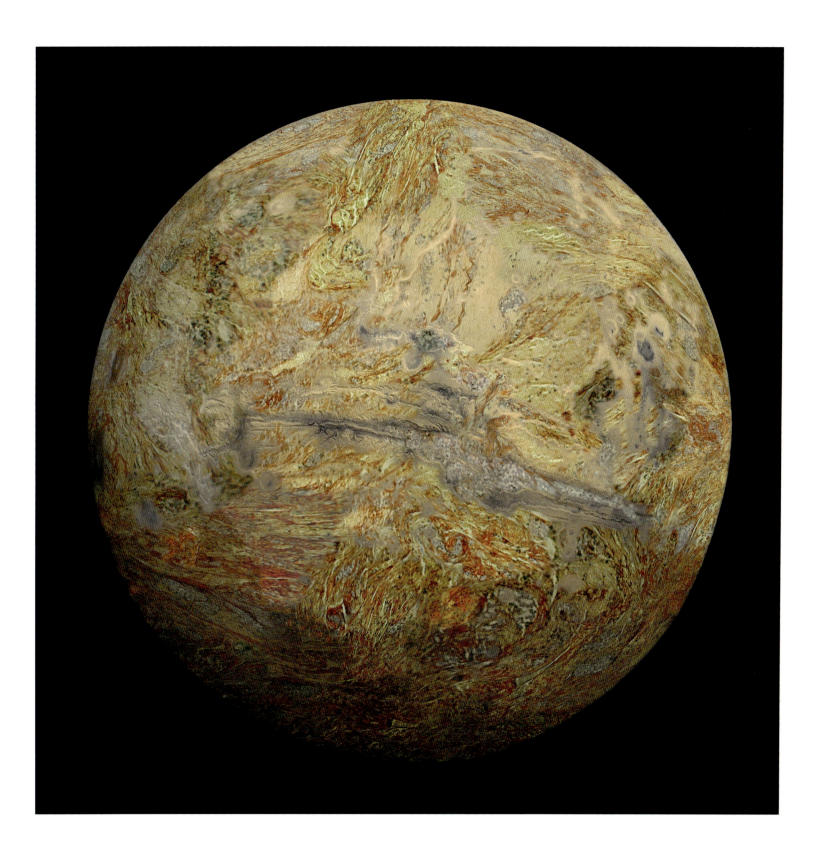

Meningo Scan

(2011)

Meninges are membranes covering the brain or spinal cord;

they are the source of brain tumors called "meningiomas".

Cells taken from an intraoperative consultation

(cytologic preparation, smear)

are rearranged in the shape of a pathology slide and surrounded

by images of many brains that might have been the source

of this type of specimen.

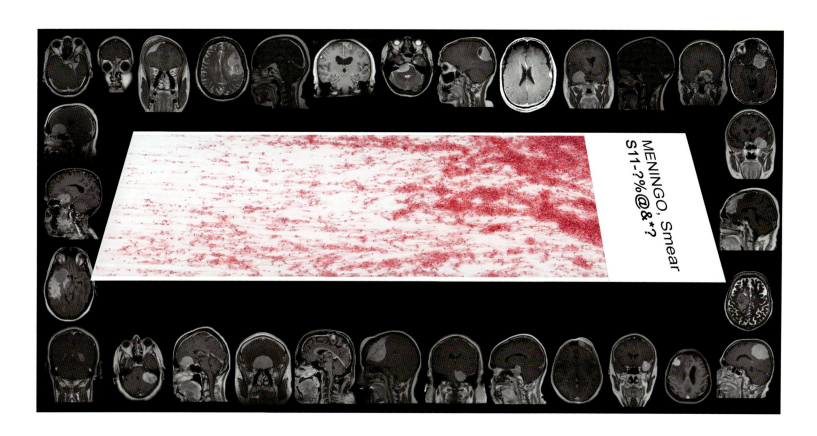

MENINGO, Smear
S11-?%@&*?

PMH in H&E

(2011)

"PMH" = Princess Margaret Hospital

"H&E" = Hematoxylin and Eosin
(the stain used routinely for histology)

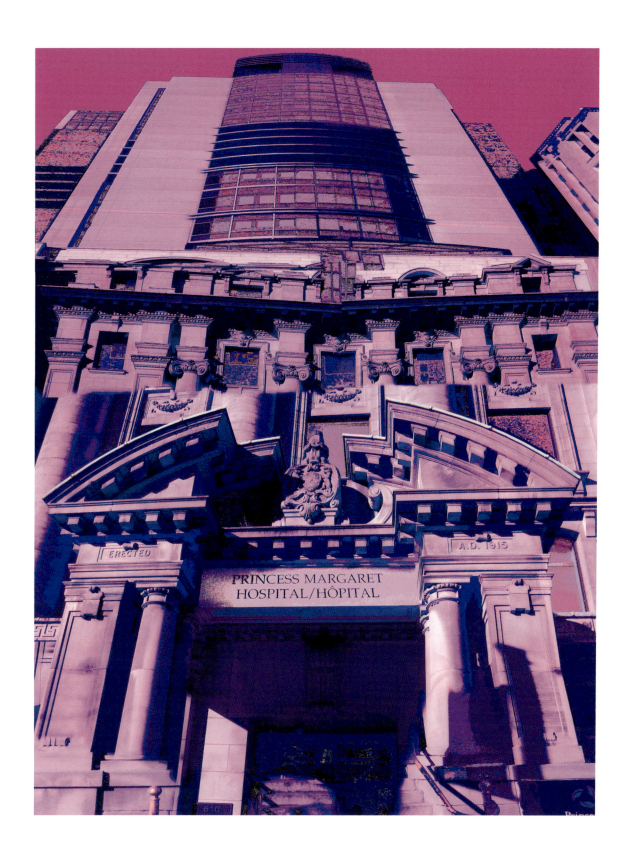

Cookie Monster Trichostasis

(2012)

Trichostasis is blockage of the hair follicle.

This hair follicle resembles the TV Muppet Cookie Monster.

(Based on microscopic images provided
by dermatopathologist Dr. Danny Ghazarian)

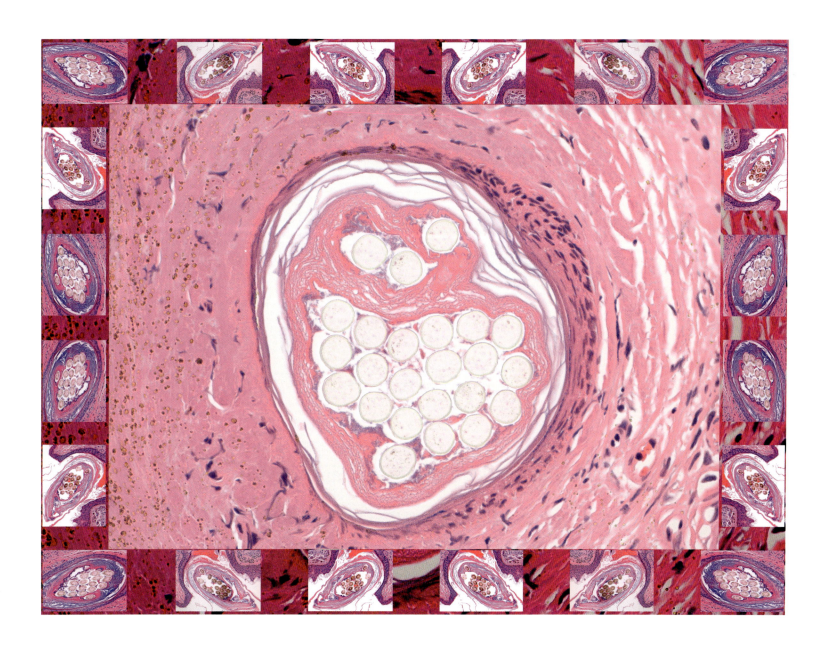

Trichoblastoma Flowers

(2012)

Trichoblastoma is a benign tumor of hair follicles.

This tumor has a beautiful pattern resembling flowers.

(Based on microscopic images provided

by dermatopathologist Dr. Danny Ghazarian)

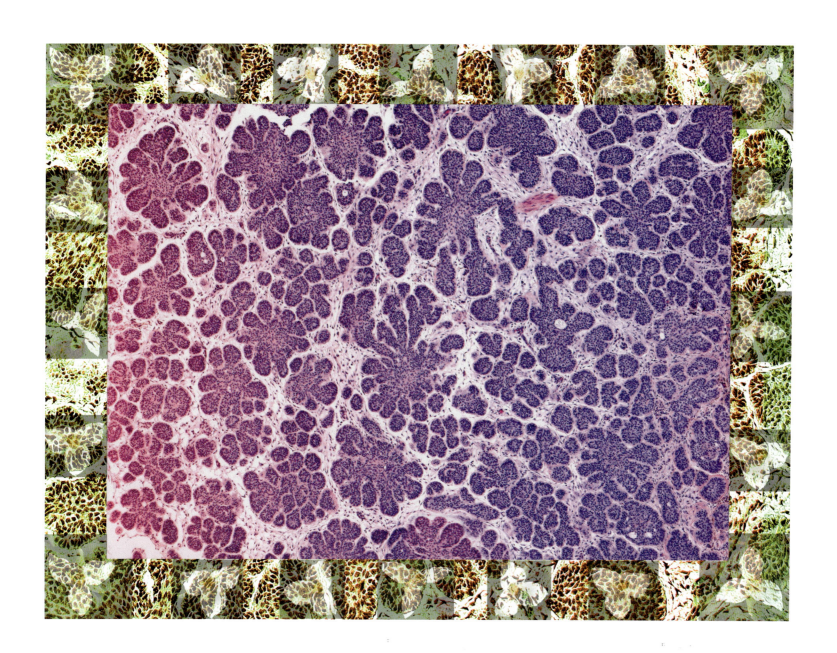

Garbage In,

Garbage Out

(2012)

In pathology, just as in computer science, flawed input

(such as mislabeled specimens, poor fixation

or low quality sectioning and staining)

results in poor quality output (diagnosis).

(some images used via CC license)

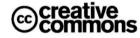

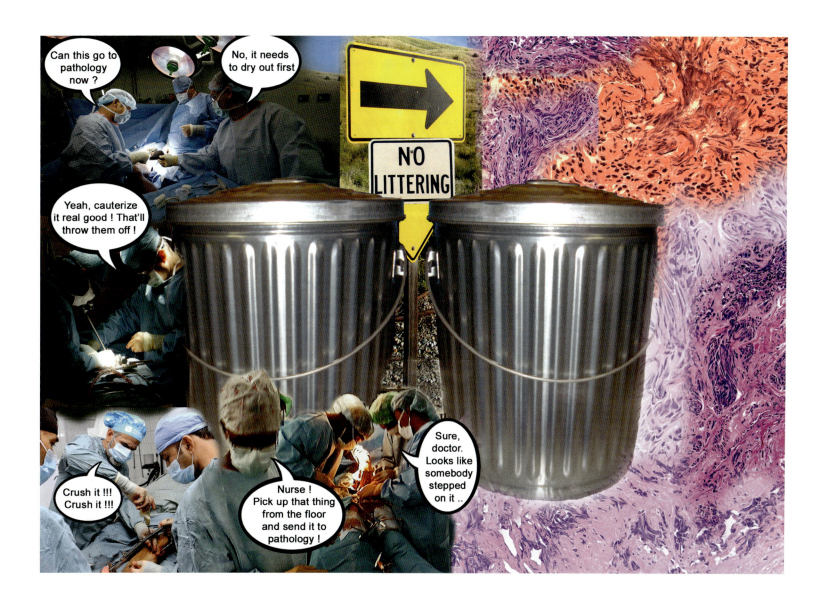

Dancing with the Star Cells

(2012)

After the famous painting "The Dance"
(La Danse) by Henri Matisse (1910).

Astrocytes (i.e. "star cells") highlighted

with immunostain for GFAP.

Colors modified for dramatic effect.

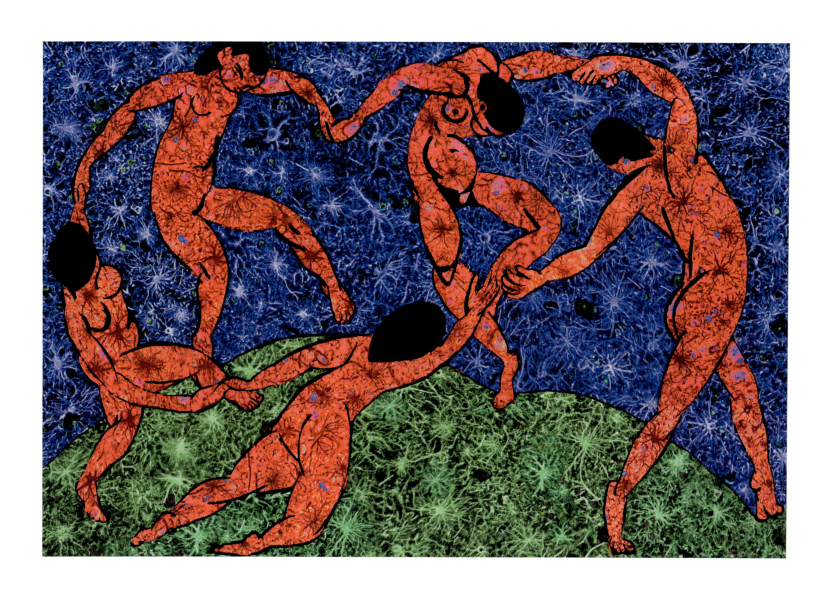

Histologic HexaQuilt

(2012)

A potpourri of histologic patterns in hexagonal shapes, combined onto a quilt-sized art piece.

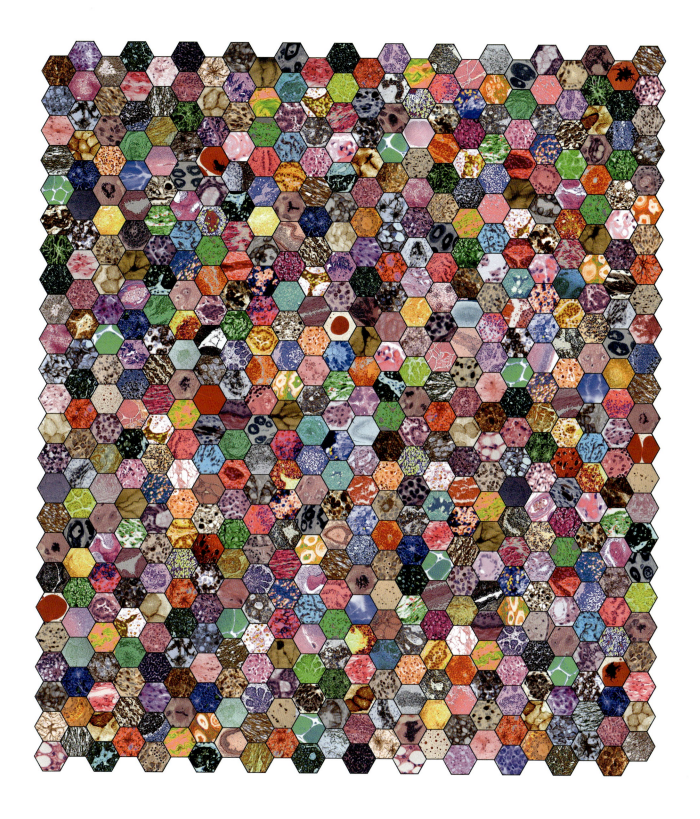

Neuropathy False Color

(2012)

From a biopsy case of a peripheral nerve.

The patient had a clinical diagnosis of peripheral neuropathy.

Color artificial-artful.

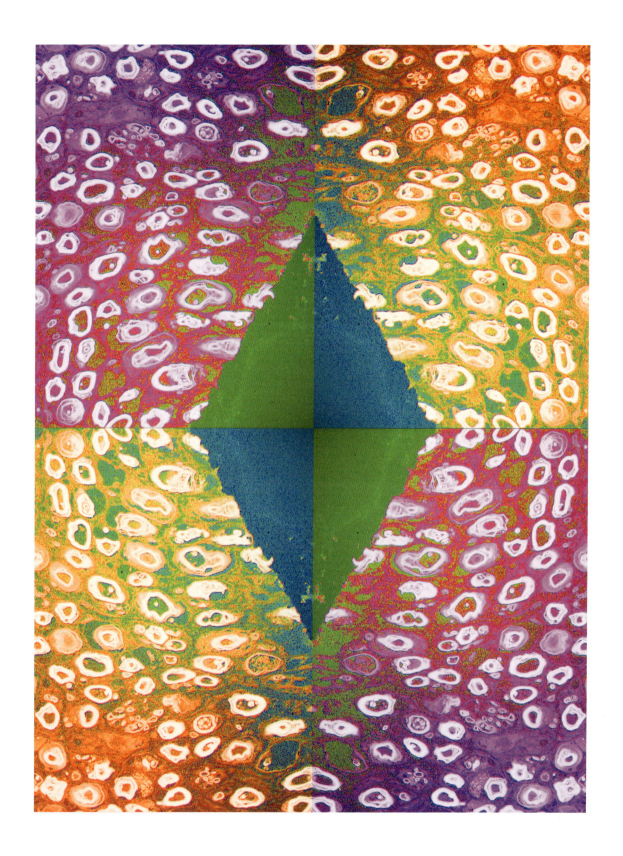

Rule Out Cancer

(2012)

Pathologists commonly receive a biopsy of a mass

with the clinical history "rule out cancer"

in the attempt to determine

whether the patient has a malignancy.

(images of ruler used via CC license)

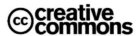

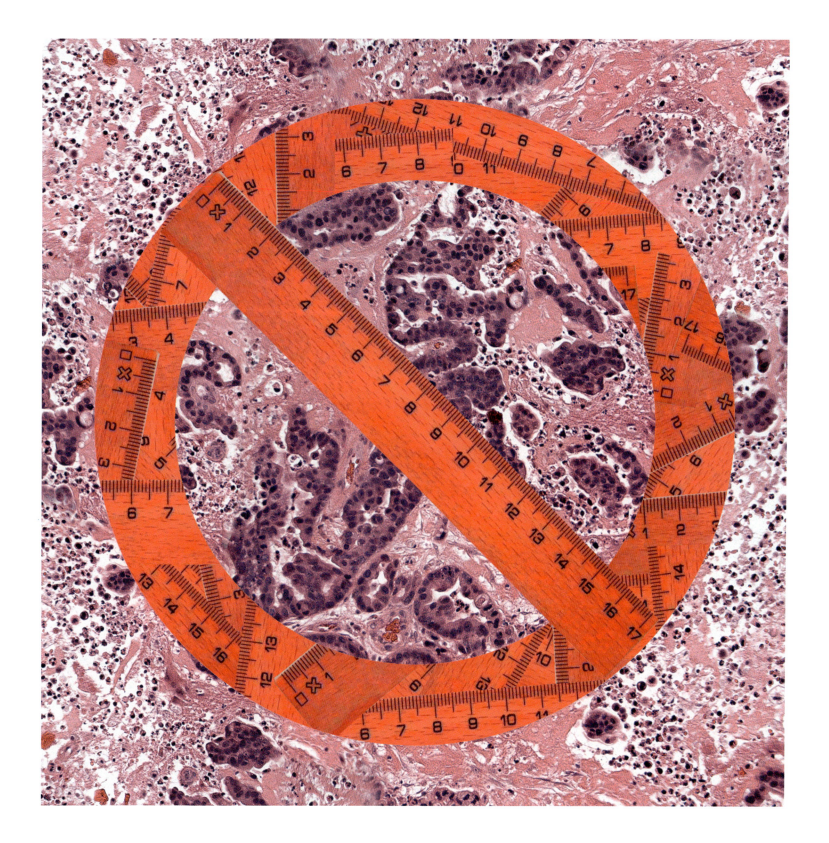

The Cancer Exploded

(2012)

High magnification of tumor cells

from a malignant brain tumor.

(images of fire from Flickr user "gynti_46", used via CC license)

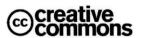

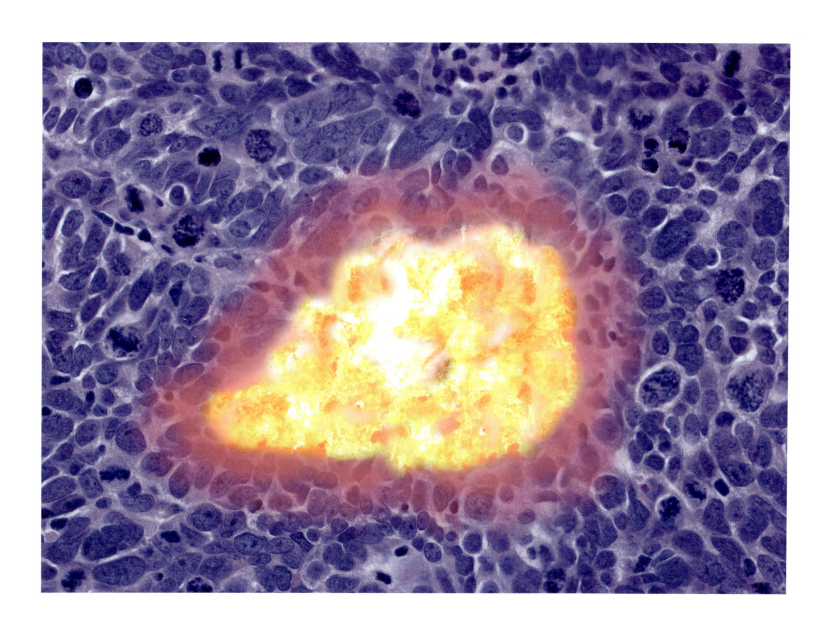

Ultrastructural Parking Lot

In many cases of mitochondrial myopathy,
electron microscopy (EM) can demonstrate so-called
paracrystalline inclusions in mitochondria,
also known as "parking lot" inclusions.

(images of parking lots used via CC license)

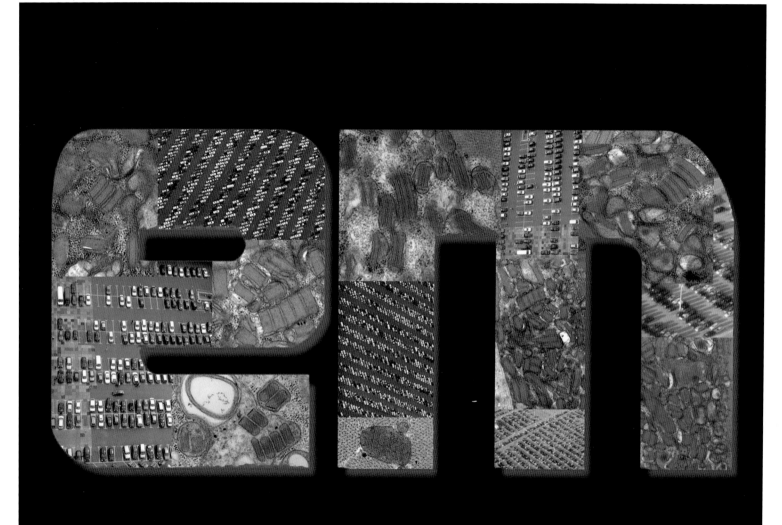

Art Gallery of Pathology

(2013)

An abstraction of the Henry Moore sculpture

in front of the

Art Gallery of Ontario in Toronto.

Original photo with multiple histologic images

from different brain and spinal tumors mapped onto it.

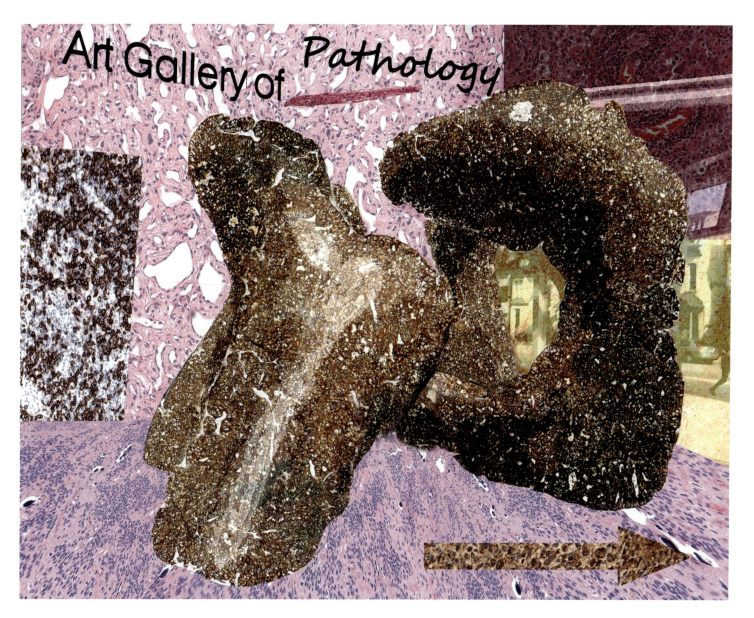

Art Gallery of Pathology

Created by Tim-Rasmus Kiehl   Edited by Sylvia L. Asa

The Great Ventricles

(2012, part of "green towel series")

Tissue sections from a brain autopsy specimen

were digitally rearranged to resemble the shape of the Great Lakes.

In the brain, the term "watershed areas"

refers to territories supplied by the main large blood vessels.

Displayed art text as follows:

"Previously described anatomic variant,

tends to occur after prolonged hypothermia (i.e. long ice age).

Watershed areas not shown."

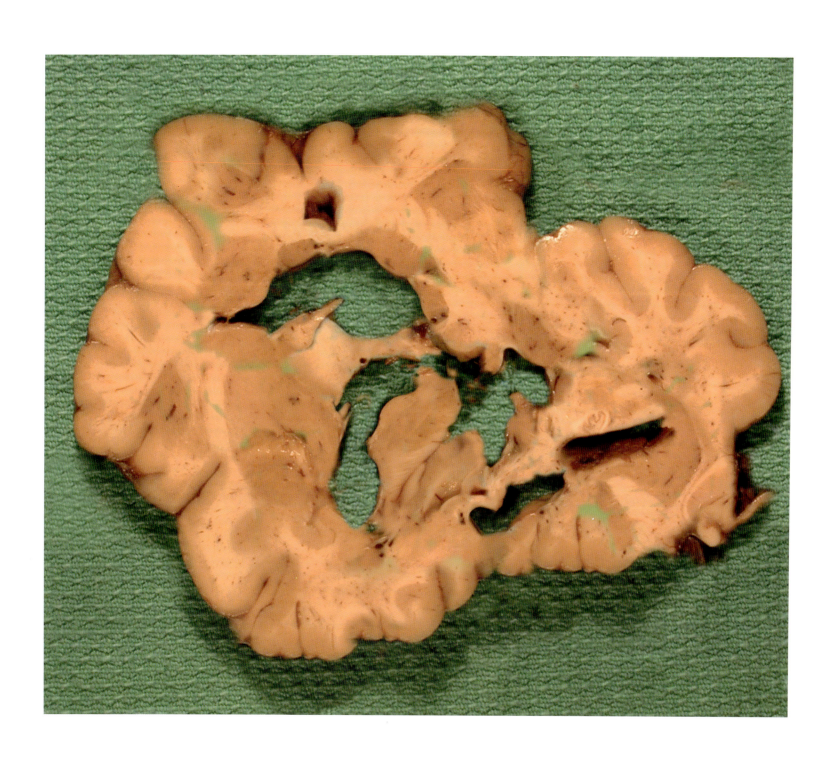

Different Strokes

(2014, part of "green towel series")

A collection of brains after sectioning, showing

the various manifestations and locations of stroke.

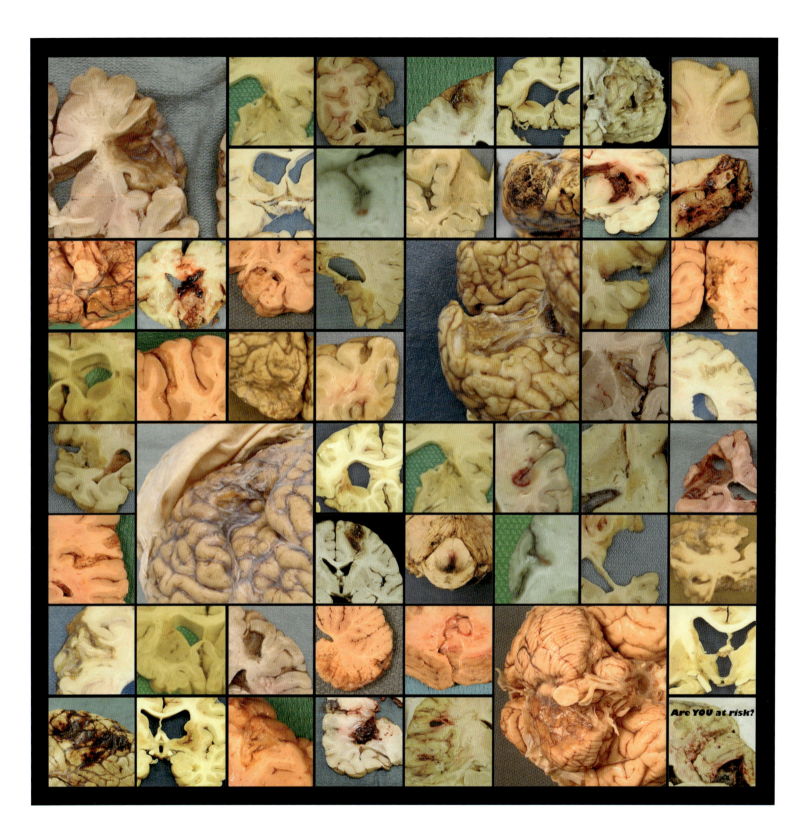

Are YOU at risk?

Pathologic Hands

(2013, part of "green towel series")

After the lithograph "Drawing Hands"
by Dutch artist M. C. Escher
that was first printed in January 1948.

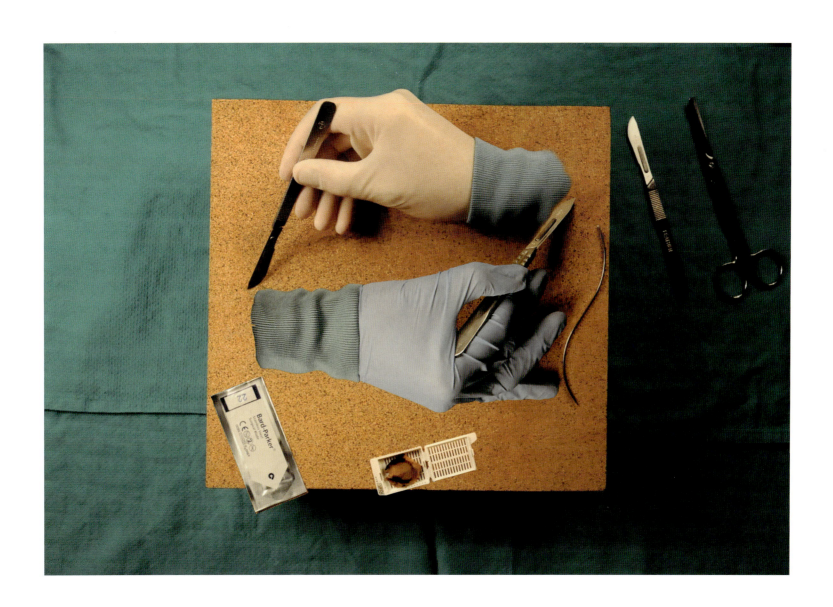

Biohazardous

(2013)

Upper left: fungus (highlighted by GMS preparation)

Upper right: bacteria (demonstrated with Gram stain)

Bottom: virus (by electron microscopy)

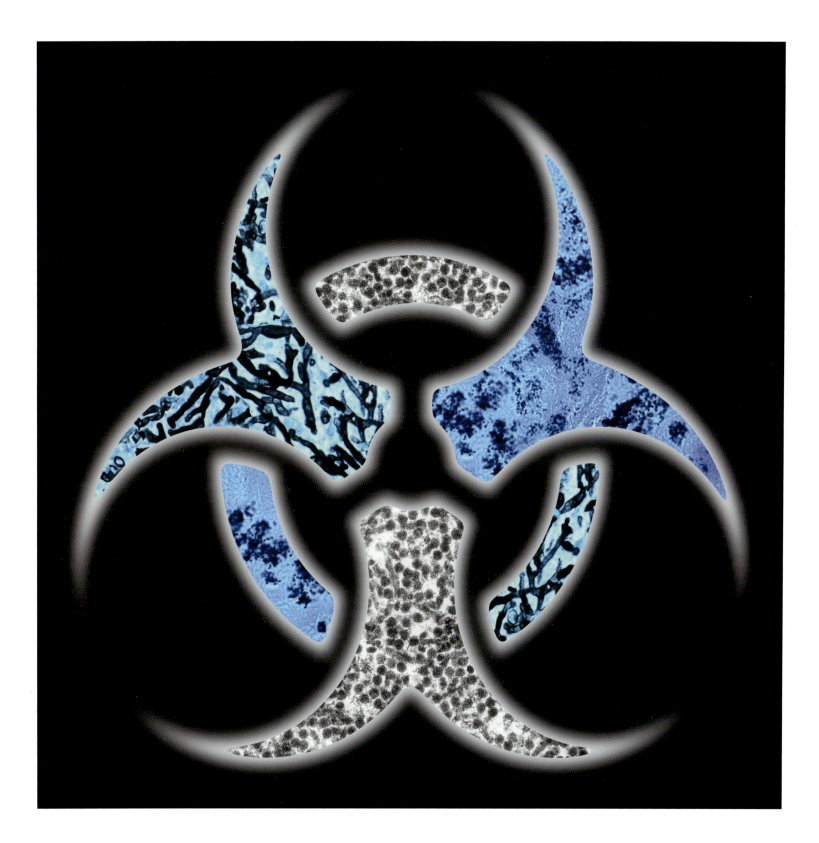

We Can Diagnose It

(2014)

Based on the American wartime propaganda poster

"We Can Do It"

by J. Howard Miller,

made in 1943 for Westinghouse Electric

as an inspirational image to boost worker morale

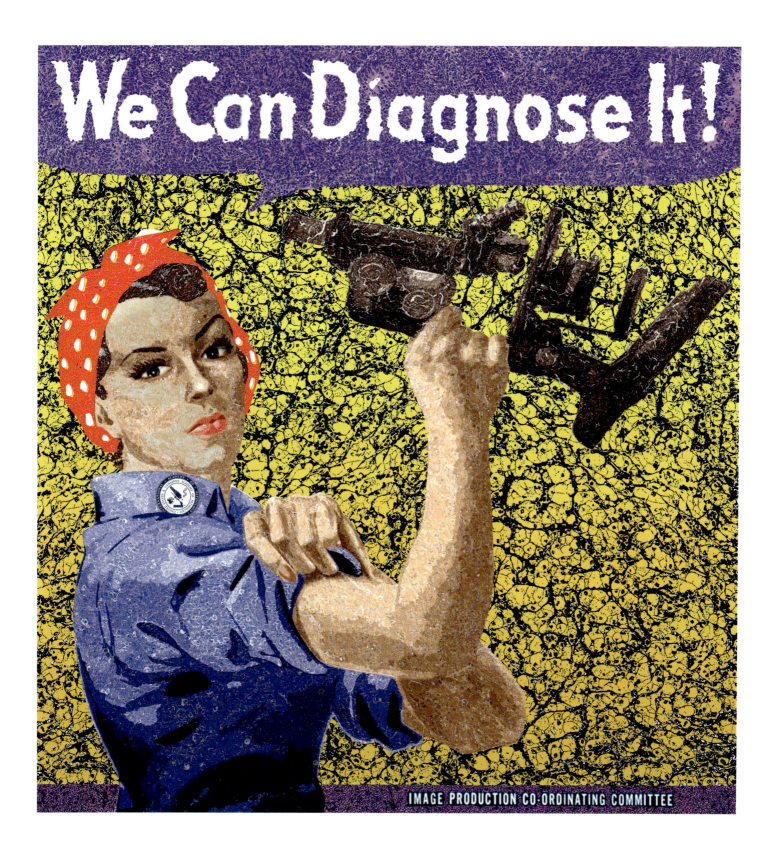

We Can Diagnose It!

IMAGE PRODUCTION CO-ORDINATING COMMITTEE

Oxytocin
Love Potion Number 1

(2015)

Oxytocin is a hormone produced by the

part of the brain known as the hypothalamus

and secreted by the posterior pituitary.

It plays a key role in loving behaviors including

pair bonding, orgasm and maternal affection.

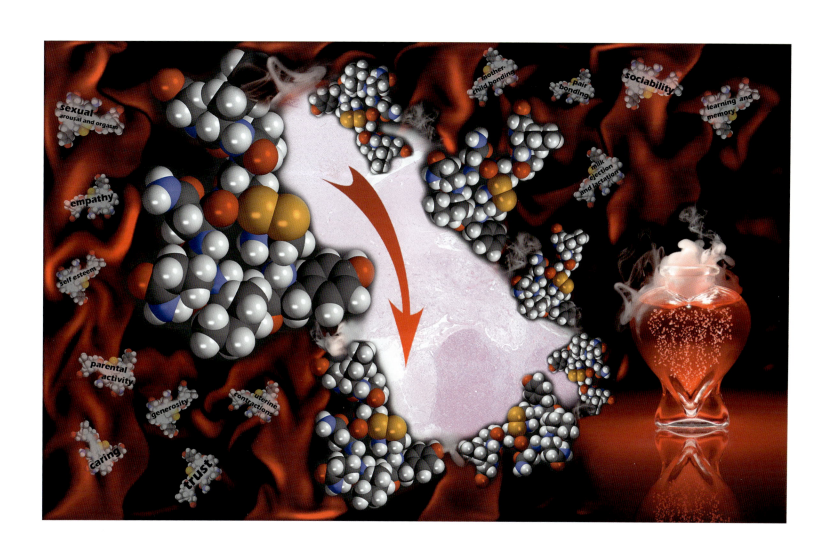

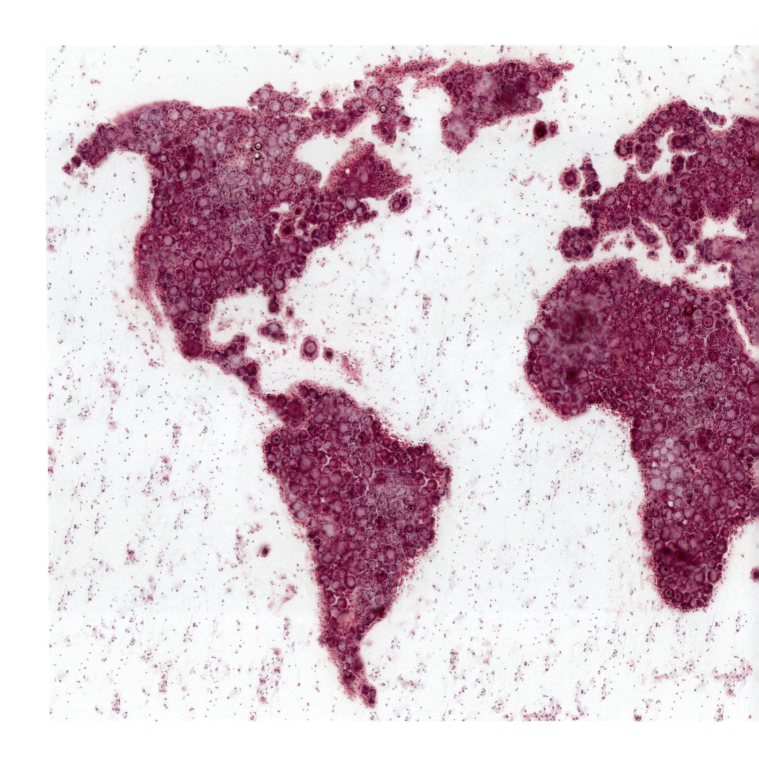

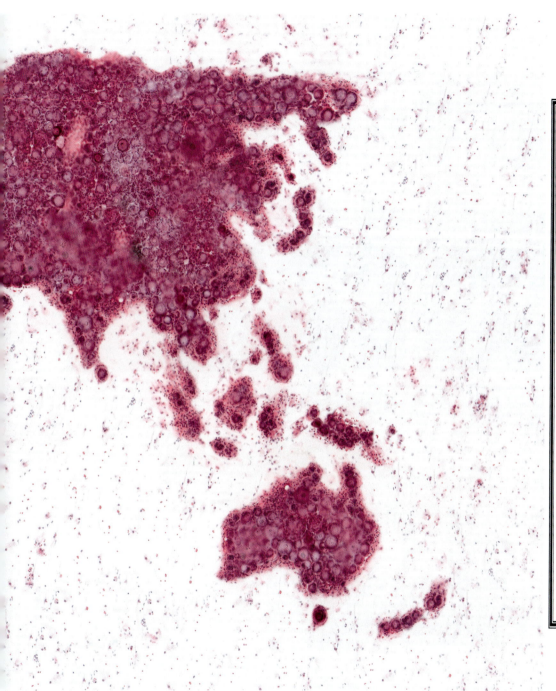

Whorl World

(2014)

This is a composite of images from an intraoperative consultation, turned into a map of the world. The source was a cytologic preparation from a meningioma, showing whorled structures and concentric microcalcifications, the so-called "psammoma bodies."

Before............

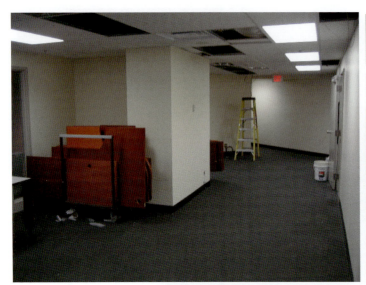 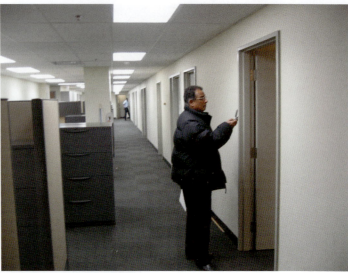

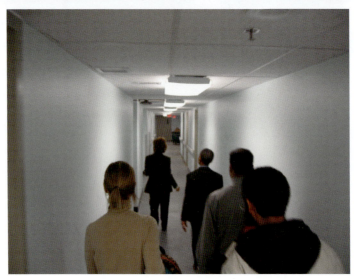

. . . . .and After

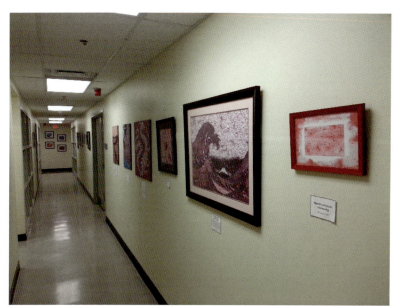

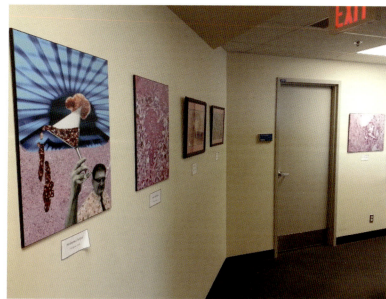

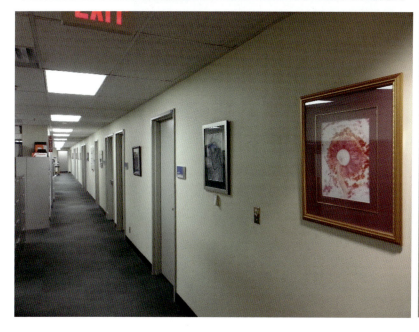

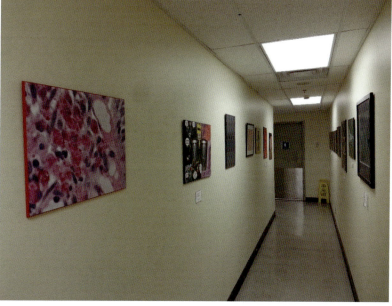

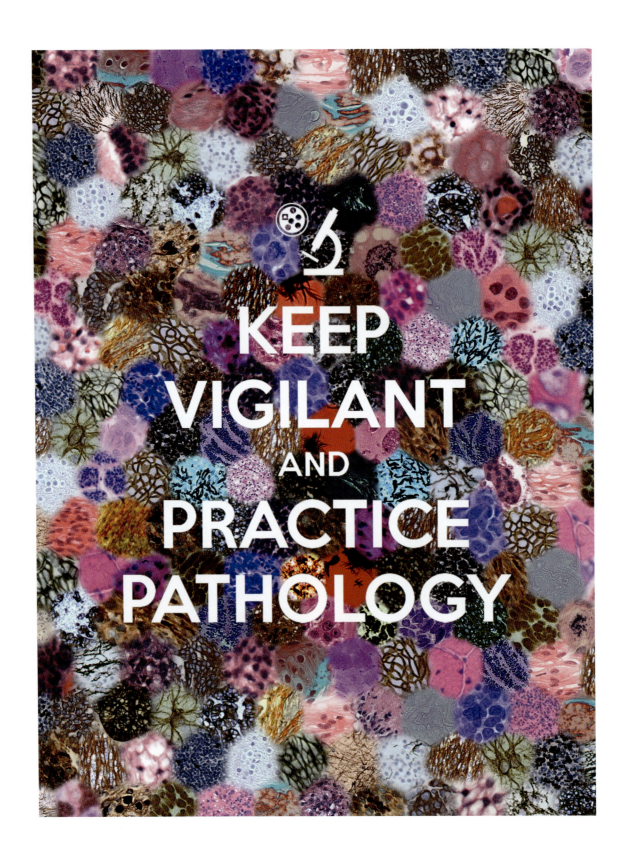